MARCHING TERMS

AND

EVOLUTIONS.

MARCHING TERMS

AND

EVOLUTIONS

BY

HERBERT E. NAYLOR

Fellow and Examiner of the Incorporated Gymnastic Teachers' Institute, London; Holder of Gymnastic Teachers' Diploma and (late) Examiner to the National Society of Physical Education, London; Diplôme Société Fédérale de Gymnastique, Switzerland; Physical Director London Central Young Men's Christian Association

WITH OVER 80 DIAGRAMS

The Naval & Military Press Ltd

Published by

The Naval & Military Press Ltd
Unit 5 Riverside, Brambleside
Bellbrook Industrial Estate
Uckfield, East Sussex
TN22 1QQ England

Tel: +44 (0)1825 749494

www.naval-military-press.com
www.nmarchive.com

In reprinting in facsimile from the original, any imperfections are inevitably reproduced and the quality may fall short of modern type and cartographic standards.

PREFACE

It has been my privilege during the past few years to examine a number of students and teachers for Gymnastic Teachers' diplomas, and nothing has impressed me more than the diversity of views displayed with regard to marching.

Whether this is due to lack of suitable text books so far as marching is concerned in voluntary gymnasia, or to the variety of terms in use at the present time, it is difficult to say, but certainly the latter has assisted to cause the confusion.

The military authorities have laid down definite formations and terms for marching, but in civilian circles the class of work is different, with a few exceptions, and requires special nomenclature to cover it.

That a definite and logical terminology is as necessary for marching as for other gymnastic exercises will doubtless be admitted, but unfortunately experts differ as to details.

To attempt to straighten matters out is a task of some magnitude, but as big efforts are frequently the outcome of minor ones, I have presumed to write the following pages in the hope that they will assist to unravel the existing state of things, and establish a definite basis for marching terms in the future.

H. E. N.

CONTENTS

	PAGE
DEFINITION OF MARCHING	1
VALUE OF MARCHING	3
PRINCIPLES OF MARCHING	4
COMMANDS	6
FALLING IN	8
TAKING DISTANCE	11
TURNS	13
NOMENCLATURE	14
VARIETIES OF MARCHING	24
PLAIN MARCHING	25
Marking Time	26
Halting	26
DOUBLE MARCHING	28
Marking Time	29
Halting	29
EXERCISES ON THE MARCH	30
Marching with Changing Step	31
Marching with Turning Left and Right About	32
Marching with Heel Raising	33
Marching with Heel Raising and Knee Bending	34
Low (or Knee Bend) Marching	35
Marching with Knee Raising	35
Marching with Knee Raising and Leg Stretching Forward	36
Hop Marching	37
Marching with Arm Raising	38
Marching with Arm Bending and Stretching	38
Marching with Arm Flinging, Parting, and Swinging	39
Marching with Combined Leg and Arm Exercises	39
FIGURE MARCHING	44
TACTICAL MARCHING	55
ORNAMENTAL MARCHING	68

MARCHING TERMS AND EVOLUTIONS.

DEFINITION OF MARCHING.

Walking and marching are sometimes confused, and although it would be difficult to lay down a hard and fast rule with regard to either, it is generally admitted that there is a great difference between them.

One frequently hears of the adage of "learning to walk before learning to run," and if walking and marching were the same, then quite a large percentage of adult persons, including gymnasts, would need to go back a few years, for it is astounding the number who do not know how to march correctly.

Etymologists inform us that *walking* is "an act of moving forward on the feet," and *marching* a "regular measured movement on foot." The latter also seems to have been connected up with the movement of troops.

These definitions at least convey something as to the difference between walking and marching, but a little amplification will perhaps assist in making the matter clearer.

Walking, as a general rule, is simply a means to an end, or, in other words, the covering of a distance on foot, while the object of marching is to cultivate uniformity of step, style, rhythmic movement, good bodily carriage, and discipline.

This does not imply that walking is devoid of the principles of marching, but rather that the special features of the latter are not imperative in the former.

VALUE OF MARCHING.

In the objects laid down on the previous page lies the value of marching, for if a person is trained in these, there is every reason to presume that that person will walk well, and judging from the slouching one is confronted with it would be difficult to over-estimate the importance of marching as a branch of physical training.

Apart from this, there is the value from the point of view of exercise. With the measured step, which ultimately produces an easy gait and co-ordinate movement, the hip, knee and ankle joints develop strength and elasticity.

It is the lack of these attributes which is responsible for the "shuffling" movements that unfortunately many young people, as well as old, have of moving forward on foot.

The question of covering long distances is also one which enters into consideration. Particularly important is it in the movement of troops, and probably this is why the word "marching" has been associated therewith in its definition.

It needs little argument to carry a decision in favour of training in marching where the movement of a large number of men over long distances is involved, as it is evident that a cultivated step and rhythmic movement will be more effective in accomplishing the task with a minimum of fatigue, than an uncontrolled and irregular action.

THE PRINCIPLES OF MARCHING.

Until recent years it was the accepted rule that marching should be performed on what is described as the "heel and toe" principle, but in many schools and gymnasia this has now been departed from and the "pointed toe" action has succeeded it.

Under the *heel and toe* method one foot is lifted forward and placed on the ground, the heel touching first, while the other heel is raised. Momentarily, therefore, the body is poised over the heel of the forward foot and the toe of the rear foot.

The weight of the body is immediately transferred forward, and the whole of the forward foot takes the weight as the rear leg swings forward with the knee slightly bent to prevent the toes touching the ground. The heel is then placed to the ground, and the movement repeated.

This action is performed by the muscles attached to the front of the thigh and pelvis contracting as the foot is brought forward, simultaneously with which the muscles at the back of the thigh attached below the knee contract and bend the knee.

During the same period the muscles of the calf of the rear leg raise the heel, and the body is tilted slightly forward.

In the *pointed toe* method the leverage and muscular action are different, as the ball of the forward foot touches the ground first. This necessitates a contraction of the muscles on the front of the thigh, also the extensors of the foot after the swinging of the leg forward.

The argument which has been put forward in favour of this form of marching is that it strengthens the arch of the foot and the knee and ankle joints. It is, in addition, considered by some to have a graceful effect, but on this and other points with regard to it there is a divergence of opinion.

Many experts are inclined to the view that it gives a "wooden" appearance to the gait, and tends to cultivate a stiffness of carriage.

As an exercise there seems to be little objection to it providing it is not carried too far, but for distance marching it has yet to prove its value.

Coupled with the leg movement in either form there is a slight swinging forward and backward of the arms. When the left leg is moving forward the right arm swings forward in unison with it, and with the right leg the left arm, thus assisting the general balance of the body.

Any cross movement of the arms should be avoided as it produces an ungainly appearance.

The carriage of the body in marching is very important. The head should be erect, and the chest well up. This does not mean that there should be any stiffness; on the contrary, the whole movement should be one of freedom, with absolute control.

COMMANDS.

The giving of commands is frequently a difficulty which causes great anxiety to a teacher. Self-consciousness is largely responsible for this, probably because it is realised that weakness in this direction will lead to defective execution of the order.

Teachers with a natural aptitude for issuing commands should consider it a valuable asset, as it is the one thing which others lack, and fail at even after long practice.

From a disciplinary point too much emphasis cannot be placed upon it, for a command should convey, not only what is required, but how the requirements are to be fulfilled, e.g. :—

If it is sharp and decisive, the movement will be of a similar nature, while if the tone of voice is somewhat lowered, and the command delivered slowly, it is an indication that the movement is to be performed slowly.

To every command there are two parts, (1) the preparatory and (2) the executive.

The first is devoted to details of the exercise; the second gives the signal for carrying the order into effect.

The preparatory portion should be as clear and as concise as possible, while the executive should be delivered in such a way as to ensure its performance in the right manner.

A pause between the two is, however, essential, and this will vary according to the class of students and the nature of the exercise.

Beginners take longer than advanced students to associate the details with the movement, and the pause should, therefore, be more lengthy in the former case than in the latter. Further, a complicated exercise requires more thought than a simple one, and the brain must be given more time for contemplation.

Much depends on the tone of voice in which the command is given. Shouting is unnecessary, and will only serve to create a noisy class, but the voice should be lifted sufficiently for everyone to hear plainly.

Monotony of voice must be guarded against, as it tends to make a lesson irksome.

The command, therefore, is of vital importance, and every teacher will do well to cultivate a good delivery.

FALLING IN.

A preliminary step to marching is "falling in," and on deciding where this is to take place, the teacher should define the spot, and give the order accordingly. Inasmuch as this can be done in "file" or in "rank," it is evident that the order should convey what is desired in this direction.

The word "file" means a body of students lined up behind each other, and "rank" a body of students lined up side by side. When the former order, therefore, is required, the command should be "In file—fall in," or the latter "In rank—fall in."

If double files or two ranks are desired, then "In double file—fall in" or "In two ranks—fall in" will be the command.

It is also advisable to have the students graduated in sizes, the shortest in front when in file formation, and on the right in rank order.

In marching the students in front decide the length of step, and if tall there is a tendency for them to make it too long, so that the short pupils behind find it difficult to keep up, whereas, with the short students in front the tall ones have simply to regulate their step to maintain an even distance.

This also improves the general appearance of the class, and facilitates the working in mass exercises, as the tall students can see over the heads of the shorter ones when demonstrations are being given.

Moreover, with certain exercises requiring human support, it is desirable to have the students as even as possible so far as height is concerned.

The military method of appointing "markers" to indicate the spot where the "falling—in" is to take place is one that is commended, viz., when the squad is required to "fall—in" in double rank the officer in command calls for the "right marker," and, placing him in position, gives the order "Fall—in." The front rank immediately takes up its position on the left of the "marker," the rear rank being two steps behind.

If the practice of graduating the sizes is adopted, the "right marker" will be the shortest student of the class, and the "left marker" the tallest. A similar arrangement can be made for "falling—in" in file, or double file.

It is also preferable where regular classes are taken to give each student a permanent number, so that the position in file, or rank, is always the same.

On taking up their positions the students should "stand at ease," that is, with the left foot about one foot length off to the left, the feet at an angle of approximately 60 degrees, and the arms hanging loosely behind, the right hand grasping the left wrist. The head should be erect, and the chest well up.

At the command "Class—attention," the left foot will be drawn smartly up to the right with the heels together, the angle of the feet being preserved, and the arms stretched down at the sides.

When in file, "Class—cover" means that the students are to get in a straight line behind the leader with a distance of about one short step between each student.

To number off the order is given, "From the front (in twos, threes, fours)—number," and as the number is called the head is turned to the right. When in double file the left file will number and the right file take the same number.

If in rank order, on "Eyes—right" all heads—with the exception of the leader on the right—will be turned to the right, and at the word "Dress" each student will get in a straight line with the leader, and by taking a series of short steps ease off until the right arm is just clear of the left arm of the student on the right. "Eyes—front" and the class will be ready to number off.

This is done on the order "From the right (in twos, threes, fours)—number." By turning the head to the left on numbering the next student is prepared somewhat, and smartness is more likely to be obtained. The head should immediately be turned to the front after numbering.

When in two ranks the rear rank will cover off the front rank, and take the same number.

The turning of the head, whether in file or rank, may be dispensed with in the case of advanced students.

TAKING DISTANCE.

In file order "Distance forward—dress" means that, with the exception of the front student, short steps are taken until, with both arms raised forward on the level of the shoulders (palms of the hands inward), the finger tips are just clear of the student in front, and the right file dressing by the left. At "Arms—down" the position of "Attention" is assumed.

In rank order it is possible to take three different distances, viz., quarter, half, and full distance. "From the right quarter distance—dress" is done by each student—except the end one on the right, who remains firm—turning the head to the right and taking short steps sideways until, by placing the right hand on the hip, the elbow is just clear of the student on the right.

"From the right, half distance—dress" is performed in a similar manner, except that the right arm is raised sideways, with the palm of the hand downward, until the finger tips clear the left shoulder of the next student, and "From the right, full distance—dress" is accomplished by taking short steps as before until, with both arms raised sideways, the finger tips just clear the finger tips of the students on each side.

In the last instance the leader raises the left arm only.

At "Arms—down" the position of "Attention" is returned to.

These distances may be taken from the "Mark—time" or during marching in a similar manner to that described.

TURNS.

From the position of "Attention" a left turn is made by pivoting smartly around to the left on the left heel and right toe and then closing the right foot up. At first it should be taught in two counts. Care is necessary that the body be turned on the first count with the heel and toe movement, or the turn has a slovenly appearance. "Right—turn" is simply the reverse of "Left—turn," and the "About—turns" are identical but for the fact that half of a complete turn is made instead of a quarter.

A "one-eighth left—turn" is half-way between the front and the left, and is performed in a similar manner to an ordinary left turn. It is sometimes termed a "half left—turn," or "left—incline," but as it is strictly only one-eighth of a complete turn the first-named command has been chosen. Its utility will be more readily recognised when considering marching terms. There are, however, many arguments which might be used in favour of the other terms.

The same principle will apply to a "one-eighth right—turn."

A "three-eighths left—turn" is half-way between a "left" and a "left about—turn." Both it and a "three-eighths right—turn" are executed on the basis of the other turns.

In all turns the arms should be kept at the sides, and not allowed to swing about.

NOMENCLATURE.

There is probably nothing more perplexing than the different terms used by various teachers in marching. One section uses "wheel," another "angle-march," and still another "file," each intending to convey the same meaning.

Even the same teachers have a habit of mixing these terms, with the result that unless the class is acquainted with them all, uncertainty as to what is required is inevitable.

Rather than accept any precedent or general nomenclature, it is proposed to endeavour to adopt a logical basis for marching terms, and with this object in view a number of illustrations have been reproduced with terms inserted below, which, apart from the fact that they have been accepted by many leading authorities, furnish a reasonable argument in their favour.

In the first place, it is presumed that the word "wheel" intends to convey the idea of a circular motion or the revolving on an axis, therefore it is difficult to reconcile a single file performing a "wheel"—or to be strictly correct a quarter wheel—when marching in the direction shown in Fig. 1. There is no circular motion, but a direct angular one, nevertheless the term "wheel" is widely used in connection with it.

Nor would the term "Angle—march" meet the

case, inasmuch as an angle march might mean an angle of 90 degrees, 45 degrees, or any other angle. But it being recognised that a " Right—turn " means a quarter turn to the right, the term " Right—file " seems to adequately fill the requirements. Moreover, it is less liable to lead to confusion when taken in conjunction with the terms for marching in rank order.

The next illustration (Fig. 2) would be expressed

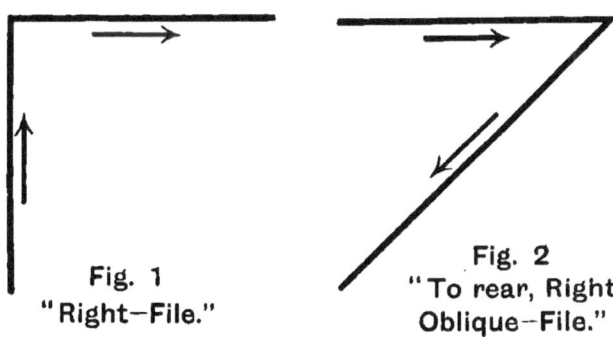

Fig. 1
"Right—File."

Fig. 2
"To rear, Right Oblique—File."

by some as " Right oblique—wheel." Assuming it is still a single file, and it being possible to march obliquely forward as well as to the rear, it is obvious that that term is unsatisfactory. It has also been quoted as an " Oblique march to the right rear," but unless there is a definite executive, the command is incomplete and must be followed by the word " march " or " forward." As every command should be as brief as possible, providing always that it is clear, "To rear, right oblique—file" meets the case much better, it being shorter and more explicit, besides preserving a suitable executive word. It should be noted here that a three-eighths right turn is made in the corner in order to file in the direction mentioned.

In Fig. 3 a three-eighths left turn is made in the corner, and "To rear, left oblique—file" is described.

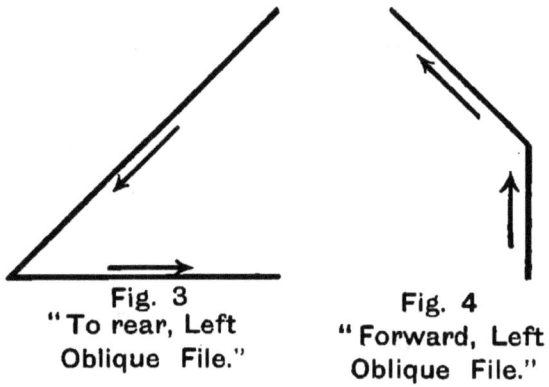

Fig. 3
"To rear, Left Oblique File."

Fig. 4
"Forward, Left Oblique File."

The necessity for showing "to rear" will be seen in the next figure (4), when only a one-eighth turn is made, and although filing obliquely the direction and angle are quite different from Figs. 2 and 3, thus the term "Forward, left oblique—file" is used.

From an oblique direction a quarter turn to the left (or right), as shown by the arrows in Fig. 5, and branching off at an angle of 90 degrees, would be "Left (or right)—file."

A whole file may make a one-eighth turn left, and march obliquely forward as in Fig. 6. This is described in military circles as "left—incline," and elsewhere as a "left oblique—march." An "incline" may mean any angle, and "left oblique—march" will be confused with filing obliquely to the left, whereas "one-eighth left—turn" will be in accordance with the ruling for a left turn, except that the latter

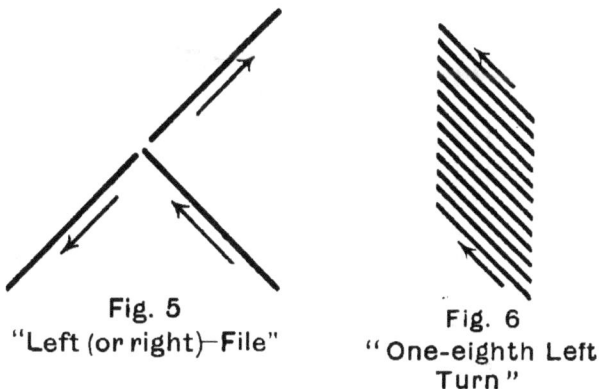

Fig. 5
"Left (or right)—File"

Fig. 6
"One-eighth Left Turn"

changes the file into a rank, and the former retains the file.

From the direction taken in Fig. 6 a further "one-eighth left—turn" would change the direction another 45 degrees left and alter the file into a rank, or a "one-eighth right—turn" would change the direction 45 degrees right (parallel to the original direction), still maintaining the file.

Fig. 7 is frequently described as a "Left about

wheel," but exception is taken to this on the ground that a squad in single file cannot wheel. It is also called a "counter march," and little objection would be made to this except that it is preferable to maintain the executive word "file" while in file formation, therefore the term "Left, counter—file."

The movement consists of filing to the left and marching in an opposite direction parallel and close to that previously taken.

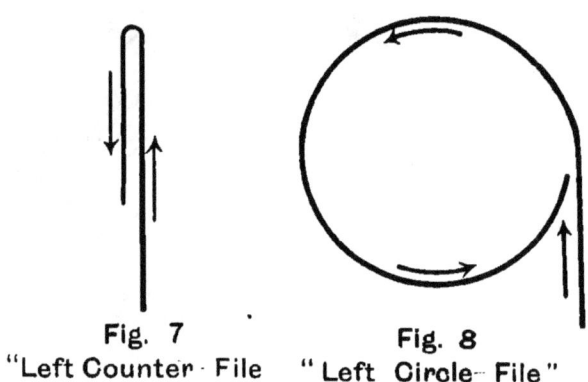

Fig. 7   Fig. 8
"Left Counter File   "Left Circle File"

It is, of course, possible to march in a circular direction as in Fig. 8, but still the action would not in any way resemble the action of a wheel, so that here the term is "(Quarter, half, three-quarters) left circle—file."

While this covers the various directions for filing, it does not deal with marching in *rank* order. This is where the term "Wheel" becomes appropriate, for its use can be justified. Whether it be ranks of two or more, when taking corners, the inside pupil forms the pivot or axis for the wheeling motion.

Study for one moment the action of the rank of four in Fig. 9. In order to manipulate the corner, the inside pupil remains on the spot making a quarter turn to the left, while the others describe a quarter wheel around him.

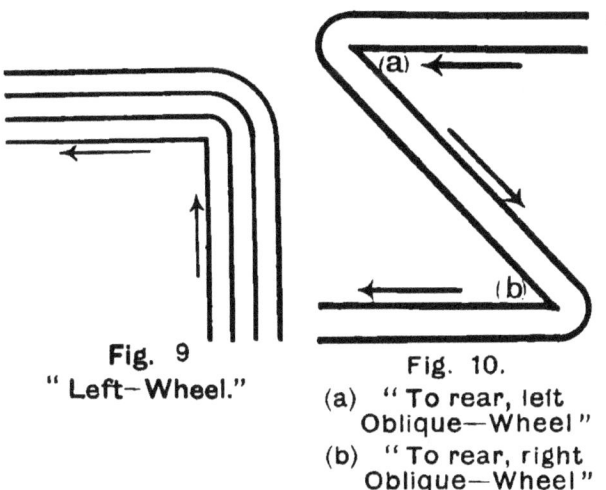

Fig. 9
"Left—Wheel."

Fig. 10.
(a) "To rear, left Oblique—Wheel"
(b) "To rear, right Oblique—Wheel"

It is practically the same action as taken by the spoke of a wheel when lying down and revolving one quarter of a circuit. Strictly, the description should be "Quarter left—wheel," but having accepted "left turn" as meaning a quarter left turn, and "left file" as an angle of 90 degrees to the left, the principle forms an unwritten law, and the word "quarter" may be omitted.

Left and right oblique wheels follow exactly the same directions as the oblique files, except that the squad being in rank order makes a wheel about an axis, while the other simply turns on a given spot. It makes no difference whether the squad is in ranks of twos as in the case of Fig. 10, as the outside pupil

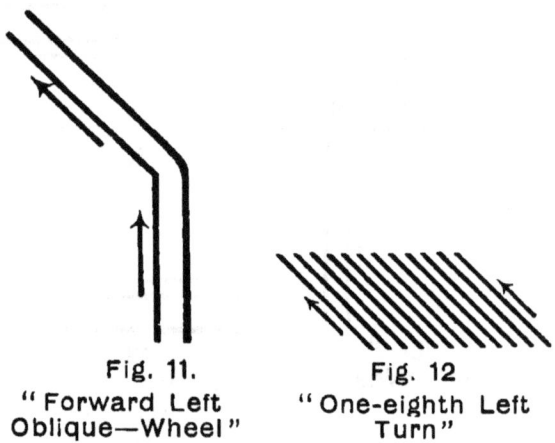

Fig. 11.
"Forward Left Oblique—Wheel"

Fig. 12
"One-eighth Left Turn"

still pivots around the inside one. It will, however, be seen that the distance covered by the outside student is greater in proportion to Fig. 9. In other words, a three-eighths wheel has been made as against a quarter.

To be consistent it might be argued that the term should be "Three-eighths left—wheel," but owing to the similarity to "To rear, left oblique—file," the term inserted is considered more suitable.

In Fig. 11 only a one-eighth wheel is made. From this it will be seen that throughout the terms for marching in ranks are identical with those for files, with the exception of the executive word of command.

To change direction of the whole rank as in Fig. 12 the command will be "One-eighth left—turn," the same principle applying as previously explained with regard to a file.

When dealing with one long rank it is sometimes desirable to make the pivot at one end of the rank, and sometimes at the other end, and a *forward* or *backward* wheel may be required. Under these circumstances a slight alteration in the command becomes necessary. For example, "Forward, quarter right—wheel" denotes a forward direction corresponding to the hands of a clock placed face upwards on the ground.

The pivot pupil is on the right, and makes a quarter right turn on the spot, while the remainder move forward a distance equal to 15 minutes on the clock, as in Fig. 13. On the other hand, "Backward, quarter right—wheel" would necessitate the pupil on the extreme left acting as a pivot and making a quarter turn to right on the spot while the remainder march backward in the direction of the hands of a clock, covering a distance equal to fifteen minutes.

For a quarter *left* wheel forward or backward the pivot student would be changed and make a quarter left turn, while the remainder would wheel around in a direction opposite to that of the hands of a clock. The "dressing" in such cases is taken from the outside, where the greatest distance is traversed and the pace set, and the pupils should touch in towards the pivot flank to avoid spaces arising in the rank.

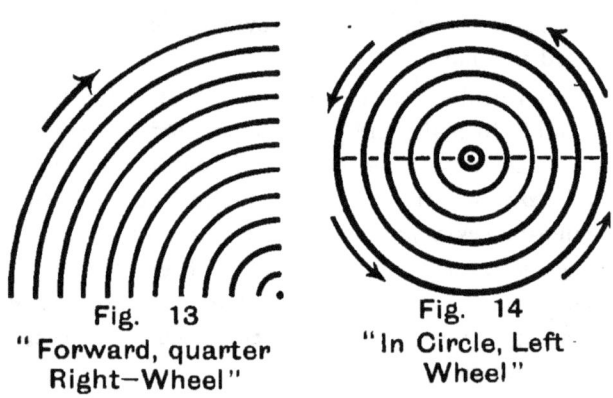

Fig. 13
"Forward, quarter Right—Wheel"

Fig. 14
"In Circle, Left Wheel"

The question next arises—What if the pivot is required in the centre of the rank, one half of the squad wheeling forward to the left, and the other half backward to the left? This certainly creates a situation not covered by any of the previous commands, but the term shown in Fig. 14, "In *circle*, left—wheel," will make a distinction, and as there is only one direction "left" there can be no misunderstanding as to which half of the squad is to go *forward* and which half *backward*.

"In *circle*, quarter left—wheel" would simply mean marching a distance equal to 15 minutes on the clock, "half" 30 minutes, and "three-quarters" 45 minutes, and if the whole circle is to be completed, then "In *circle*, left—wheel" would be the command.

The word "quarter" may be dispensed with, if desired, on the same ground as previously laid down, but this will necessitate the word "complete" being inserted in the command for a whole wheel.

One or two supplementary terms will be found necessary when taking "Figure," "Tactical," and "Ornamental" marching, but these are referred to in the special marching under those headings.

VARIETIES OF MARCHING.

Various forms of marching may be introduced without interfering with the principles already laid down, but having different objects in view, while others deviate from those principles, although they are still included in the category of marching. The following headings have, therefore, been selected:—

>PLAIN MARCHING.
>DOUBLE MARCHING.
>EXERCISES ON THE MARCH.
>FIGURE MARCHING.
>TACTICAL MARCHING.
>ORNAMENTAL MARCHING.

PLAIN MARCHING.

This consists of ordinary marching between given points. Slight changes in formation may be permitted, but generally speaking, the original formation is maintained, and any change in direction is made without having as its object the introduction of the other specified forms of marching.

Naturally, plain marching is the first stage of marching, and should be accomplished with some degree of accuracy before the more complicated types are introduced.

The main features of such marching have already been explained, but there are a number of points which need to be noted.

For example, to ensure uniformity, it is always necessary to commence with the left foot, and maintain a regular pace and time. The question arises— What is the recognised pace and time?

In the first place, it is advisable to sub-divide the heading into "Slow" and "Quick" marching, with regard to which certain authorities state that for the former the pace should be 30 inches, and the time 75 to a minute, and the latter a similar pace at 120 to a minute.

It will readily be seen that a boy of 4 feet 6 inches in height will take a shorter step than a man of 6 feet, but dealing relatively with the time there will be no material difference. Therefore, if the number of paces to the minute is agreed for "slow" and "quick" marching, it is only a question of length of pace where a disparity will be found, and this can easily be adjusted to the requirements of the situation as it presents itself.

In a "slow" march the ankle and knee are stretched as the leg swings forward so that the ball of the foot touches the ground first.

The commands are "Slow—march" or "Quick—march," as the case may be. When in rank this should be prefixed with the caution "By the right (left)" to direct the dressing.

MARKING TIME is associated with marching, but differs in that there is no movement forward. It is accomplished by a slight raising of the knees—alternately left and right—at the same time the ankle is stretched so that the toes point downward. The foot only leaves the ground a few inches, and when it is placed down the ball of the foot precedes the remaining part. The command is "Mark—time."

HALTING from the march or marking time is usually performed to two counts. From the march, the final step is completed on "one," and the rear foot closed up on "two." If marking time, two further movements are made, the conclusion being denoted by a slight emphasis with the foot on the second count.

Some teachers prefer the finish to be practically simultaneous with the executive word of the command, or only one count is allowed for the finish, but this is not very satisfactory as there are usually a number of students whose mental powers are insufficiently sensitive to grasp the order and put it into effect quickly enough, with the result that irregularity ensues.

Others take a further extreme by awaiting for the right foot to be on the ground before giving the executive word "Halt." This leads to unnecessary delay, and when it is particularly desired to bring a squad to a standstill quickly the result is unsatisfactory. The command is "Class—halt.

DOUBLE MARCHING.

Double marching is to running what ordinary marching is to walking. Running may be a means to an end, whereas double marching has a specific object, viz., the development of agility, the stimulation of the heart and lungs, and the training of the latter to accommodate their action to the muscular movement. The general effect on the bodily system is exhilarating, and the power of endurance is improved.

As the term "double" indicates the time is practically twice as fast as for ordinary marching, and by reason of the action the step is also much longer. A further feature is that double marching is performed entirely upon the toes, the body being propelled through space by a series of leaps from each foot. Only one foot touches the ground at a time, and during the remaining part of the movement the body is poised in the air. In consequence of the speed and the amount of work involved in lifting the body, the muscular action is necessarily strong, but by manipulating the weight and the bodily levers the movement is materially assisted.

For this reason the body is inclined slightly forward, and the arms—with a bend at the elbows and the hands lightly clenched—are swung freely from the shoulders. Owing to the fact that after the strong contraction of the muscles of the thigh and pressure of the foot from behind the body is lifted from the ground, it is unnecessary to bend the leg as it is swung forward, except just sufficiently to break the force of the landing.

The command is " Double—march."

DOUBLE MARKING TIME is practically a repetition of the double march action except that there is no movement forward. The leaps being made on the same spot does away with the necessity of inclining the body forward, although the bend of the knees is more accentuated.

The command is " Double mark—time."

HALTING from the " Double march " or " Double mark—time " is usually performed to four counts owing to the quick nature of the exercise. The first three counts are used for slowing down, and the final for the halt. It may be taken to a lesser number of counts, but uniformity of finish is not so easily secured.

On the other side it may be argued that the additional steps may be inconvenient when it is desired to stop suddenly.

Placed against the advantages of a smart finish this claim is scarcely likely to take preference, as the difference in distance is not very appreciable.

To change from " Double—march " to " Quick—march " the command is " Change into, quick—march," and vice versa from the " Quick—march " to the " Double—march."

EXERCISES ON THE MARCH.

A great variety of exercises may be introduced while on the march, but as previously stated no attempt should be made in this direction until a degree of proficiency has been reached in plain marching.

The exercises here set forth do not by any means form a complete list, but they allow of fifty or more changes, and with a little initiative on the part of teacher, additions and alterations can be made which will further widen the scope of their utility.

It is not suggested that they should be taken in the order placed, as they have been divided into three groups, viz. :—

Leg exercises.
Arm exercises.
Combined leg and arm exercises.

The first two of the leg series take their priority owing to the liability of their being called early into use. They are not so easy as some of the exercises which follow them, but are decidedly more important, and for this reason have been given precedence.

With regard to the remaining exercises it is recommended that an easy leg movement be followed by an easy arm movement, and when a number of such exercises have been acquired the easier combinations may be attempted. The combinations should not, however, be taken unless the general ability of the students justifies it, as it is unwise to overtax the powers of pupils.

MARCHING WITH CHANGING STEP.

It frequently happens that beginners, and sometimes advanced students, get out of step, and unless they have been taught how to get into step again confusion ensues.

An exercise, therefore, embodying the changing of step not only tends to develop control, but gives confidence in circumstances such as mentioned.

To accomplish the change, the rear foot makes a short, quick step so that the instep is close to the heel of the forward foot, upon which the forward foot immediately advances a further step, the two movements being made to one ordinary count, and the rear foot follows in the usual manner, thereby resuming ordinary marching.

When this has been practised a few times with either foot forward, and to the command " Change—step," it may be carried out at every fourth step, or any number of steps that may be decided, and finally a succession of changes with each foot will afford sufficient opportunity for becoming proficient in this step.

Changing step while " Marking—time " is carried out by remaining firmly on one foot while the other makes two taps on the ground at ordinary time, then resuming as before.

MARCHING WITH TURNING LEFT AND RIGHT ABOUT.

Turning about on the march is a difficult exercise, and requires considerable practice before being satisfactorily performed, yet, when surveying the movements comprising it, there does not seem anything to account for this difficulty.

Possibly the explanation lies in the fact that the intellects of some pupils do not respond as quickly as others. Certainly the succession of events in turning about on the march follow each other quickly, and call for some amount of mental alertness.

Spread over four counts "Right about—turn" is given when the left foot is forward. At "one" and "two" the left and right feet each make a further step forward. At "three" the right about turn is made on the toes, and at "four" the left foot swings forward, taking the first step in the opposite direction. "Left about—turn" is given when the right foot is forward, and the above movements are reversed. In teaching this exercise it is advisable to start from a stationary position with the left or right foot forward, and then carry out the movements by numbers slowly.

In military circles "About—turn" means "Right about—turn," and the first, second, and third motions are executed on place, the left foot moving forward on the fourth count.

MARCHING WITH HEEL RAISING.

This exercise consists of raising the heels while on the march. At "Heels—raise" the knees should be pressed well back, and the ankle stretched to full extent. The step is naturally shortened, and the movement is somewhat a stiff one, but it is useful for strengthening the arch of the foot.

It may be carried out with the arms swinging freely at the sides, or they may be kept rigid. At "Class—halt," the leg moving forward should complete its step (one) and the rear foot drawn up (two), both heels being lowered on the second count.

With advancement the hands may be placed on the hips, the arms bent upwards, forward, in "neck rest" position, stretched forward, sideways, or upward.

When these combinations are made the command should be given, " With heels raising, hips—firm," or " With heels raising, arms upward—bend," the order being performed immediately on the executive word " firm " or " bend," etc. To resume ordinary marching the method of returning the arms to the sides should be named, e.g., " With heels lowering, arms downward—stretch."

To "halt" from the combined position the order will be " With arms stretching downward, class—halt," or " With arms swinging downward (forward

D

and downward, sideways and downward), class—halt."

If there are two movements of the arms one will be made on each count, and if only one on the second count, so as to finish with the leg movement.

MARCHING WITH HEEL RAISING AND KNEE BENDING.

Before attempting heel raising and knee bending on the march, it should be performed from the stationary position, and when this has been satisfactorily accomplished it may be done at every fourth step, or according to requirements. Four counts are necessary to complete it.

At "one" the heels are raised, "two" the knees bent until the thighs are at right angles to the legs (knees turned well out), "three" the knees are stretched, and "four" the heels lowered. When on the march, and the order is given, "At every fourth step, heel raising and knee bending—begin," the next step after the executive word counts "one"; three further steps are then taken to "two," "three," and "four," and on the next count the rear foot is drawn up, both heels being raised to make the first movement of the exercise, the remaining three being as hitherto explained. On the completion of the exercise, the next four steps are made, and the whole is repeated as desired. The stepping forward after the heel raising and knee bending is done alternately with left and right foot.

LOW (OR KNEE BEND) MARCHING.

From the knee bend position in the last exercise the march may be continued by taking short, slow steps forward on the toes.

It is a difficult exercise, as it requires a fair amount of balance, in addition to which its muscular action is very strong. When taken from a stationary position, the order is given as for "Heel raising and knee bending," and then "Forward—march." "Class—halt" is made to four counts, a further step forward being taken on "one," the rear foot drawn up on "two," the knees stretched on "three," and the heels lowered on "four."

If "Low march (or knee bend march)—change" is given during ordinary marching, the knee bend position is immediately assumed.

MARCHING WITH KNEE RAISING.

Knee raising while on the march is done to slow march time, and the step is slightly shorter than the ordinary march step. If starting from the position of "Attention," the command is "With knee raising, forward—march," and the left knee is raised until the thigh is at right angles to the trunk, the leg being perpendicular, forming a further right angle to the thigh, and the ankle stretched.

The leg is then smartly stretched forward and downward, the ball of the foot meeting the ground first. Simultaneously with the stretching of the leg the weight of the body is thrown forward, and the heel of the rear foot raised.

This action is repeated with the rear leg, and continued until "Class—halt" or "Change—march" is given, when the moving leg completes its action and the rear foot is drawn up, or ordinary marching is resumed.

To change from ordinary marching the order is given "With knee raising change—march," the moving foot then completes the next step forward and the rear knee is raised. Marking time with knee raising differs only from ordinary marking time in that the knees are raised higher.

MARCHING WITH KNEE RAISING AND LEG STRETCHING FORWARD.

The only difference between this exercise and the preceding one is that following the knee raising the leg is stretched forward, instead of forward and downward, and a further count is taken to lower it to the ground. The balance effect of the movement is stronger than in the "knee raising" exercise. The same rules as for the former exercise apply to halting.

HOP MARCHING.

Plain hopping consists of raising one leg in the rear and taking a series of short leaps on the ball of the other foot. Attention to the bodily carriage is very essential in this exercise. The head should be erect with the chin drawn in, the chest well up, and the raised leg straight with the knee and ankle joints stretched.

Great variety may be introduced by hopping a stipulated number of steps on one foot, and then changing on to the other and performing a similar number on that foot, or by interspersing the hopping with marching steps.

Hopping alternately on the left and right foot provides further opportunities for variety, the raising of the leg in the rear being slightly accentuated with each hop. The leg or the knee may also be raised forward during the hop.

The commands for these exercises will be :—

"On the left (right) foot—hop."

"With two (three, four) steps left and right foot alternately—hop."

"With three steps hop and three steps march—hop."

"With leg (knee) raising forward—hop."

"With leg (knee) raising forward left and right foot alternately—hop."

The hopping will begin from the named foot on the completion of the next ordinary step after the order has been given. It is advisable to place the hands on the hips or in some other steady position during these exercises, unless combined with arm movements.

MARCHING WITH ARM RAISING.

Arm raising on the march may be executed forward, sideways, forward and upward, and sideways and upward. In the last two instances the return may be either forward and downward, or sideways and downward. Any number of counts can be allotted, but at first it is recommended to be taken to four.

Thus, "With arm raising, forward—march," (1) the left foot moves forward and the arms are raised; (2) the right foot moves forward, the arms remaining in position; (3) the left foot moves forward and the arms return to sides; (4) the left foot moves forward while the arms remain at the sides.

Several combinations of the arm movements are possible by extending the number of counts, e.g., (1) raise arms forward, (2) retain position, (3) raise arms upward, (4) retain position, (5) lower arms sideways, (6) retain position, (7) lower arms downward, (8) retain position.

MARCHING WITH ARM BENDING AND STRETCHING.

The exercises under this heading need little explanation after the remarks with regard to arm raisings. The bend is made on the first count, and the stretch on the third. The simple stretching forward, sideways, and upward, should be taken separately at the beginning. Combinations of these will permit of quite advanced exercises, such as, one arm being stretched in one direction while the other is stretched in another. The commands will follow the same principle as described hitherto.

MARCHING WITH ARM FLINGING, ARM PARTING, AND ARM SWINGING.

Exercises in this group are carried out in exactly similar methods to those under arm raising and arm stretchings.

MARCHING WITH COMBINED LEG AND ARM EXERCISES.

It is not proposed to go into details of the various combinations permitted under this heading, as a large number of them will be apparent both in regard to the exercise and the method of execution. Only a general outline is given, therefore, with a few explanatory notes at the end.

1.—Heels raising with arm raisings.

2.—Heels raising with arm bendings and stretchings.

3.—Heels raising with arm flingings, partings, and swingings.

4.—Heel raising and knee bending with arm raisings.

5.—Heel raising and knee bending with arm bendings and stretchings.

6.—Heel raising and knee bending with flingings, partings, and swingings.

7.—Knee bending (low march) with arm raisings.

8.—Knee bending (low march) with arm bendings and stretchings.

9.—Knee bending (low march) with arm flingings, partings, and swingings.

10.—Knee raising with arm raisings.

11.—Knee raising with arm bendings and stretchings.

12.—Knee raising with arm flingings, partings, and swingings.

13.—Knee raising and leg stretching forward with arm raisings.

14.—Knee raising and leg stretching forward with arm bendings and stretchings.

15.—Knee raising and leg stretching forward with arm flingings, partings, and swingings.

16.—Hopping with arm raisings.

17.—Hopping with arm bendings and stretchings.

18.—Hopping with arm flingings, partings, and swingings.

Explanatory Notes.

1 to 3.—The arm movements are performed the same as in ordinary marching.

4.—The arm raisings are taken with the heels raising, held during the knee bending and stretching, and returned when the heels are lowered. Thus the arms move on the first and fourth counts.

5.—The arms are bent on the first count with the heels raising, stretched on the second count with the knee bending, bent again on the third count with the knee stretching, and stretched downward to attention on the fourth count with the heels lowering.

6.—One movement of the arms is taken to each count of the heels raising and knee bending, as in No. 5.

7 to 9.—The arm movements are performed the same as in ordinary marching.

10.—The arms are raised with the knee and lowered as the leg is stretched forward and downward.

11.—The arms are bent with the knee raising, and stretched with the leg stretching forward and downward.

12.—One movement of the arms accompanies the knee raising and another the leg stretching.

13.—The arms take up the first position to the knee raising, hold it during the leg stretching forward, and are lowered when the foot is placed to the ground.

14.—When the knee is raised the arms are bent, and when it is stretched the arms are stretched, the latter remaining in position during the third count.

15.—The rhythm of exercises in this group will be better maintained by taking up the first position of the arms with the knee raising, holding it during the knee stretching, and flinging, parting, or swinging on the third count when the leg is lowered.

16 to 18.—If a succession of hops are being made on one foot, the arm raising (bending, swinging) should be executed on the first hop, held during the second, lowered (stretched, flung, parted, swung) on the third, and kept steady during the fourth. When hopping left and right alternately, the first position is taken to the hop on the left foot, and the second to the hop on the right foot.

So far as the commands for these exercises are concerned, the following will form a guide for the whole:—

1 to 3.—" With heels raising and arms stretching upward, forward—march."

4 to 6.—" With heel raising and knee bending, combined with arm flinging, forward—march."

7 to 9.—" With arms swinging forward and upward, low—march."

10 to 12.—" With knee raising and arms stretching sideways, forward—march."

13 to 15.—" With knee raising and leg stretching forward, combined with arms parting, forward—march."

16 to 18.—" With arms swinging sideways and upward, on left and right foot alternately—hop."

If it is desired to change from ordinary marching into any of these exercises it will be necessary to replace the word "forward," preceding the executive word "march," by the word "change," e.g., "With heels raising and arms stretching upward, change—march."

FIGURE MARCHING.

A very wide scope presents itself under this heading as innumerable shapes and forms can be adopted. Stars, crosses, diamonds, crescents, squares, outlines of letters, numerical figures, and, in fact, marching in any distinct outline may be included in this category.

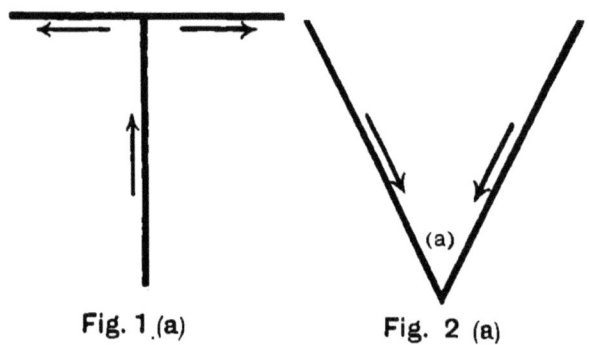

Fig. 1 (a)   Fig. 2 (a)

Of the more simple types the following are a few examples (the terms used are those dealt with in the chapter on " Nomenclature ") : —

Beginning with a single file marching in the direction of the arrow of Fig. 1 (a), " Left and right, alternately—file " will make a letter " T."

" To rear, left and right oblique—file " to the point (a), the first leader at (1) taking the first command will form a letter " V " (Fig. 2 (a)).

The leaders being at the apex of the "V," the order "Forming single file, to rear, left and right—file" will take them along the middle line, and when in the centre "Forward, left and right alternately oblique—file" will form a letter "Y" (Fig. 3 (a)).

Continuing further the top part of this letter will make the inside lines of the letter "M" (Fig. 4 (a)). "To rear, left and right oblique—file" will then complete the letter.

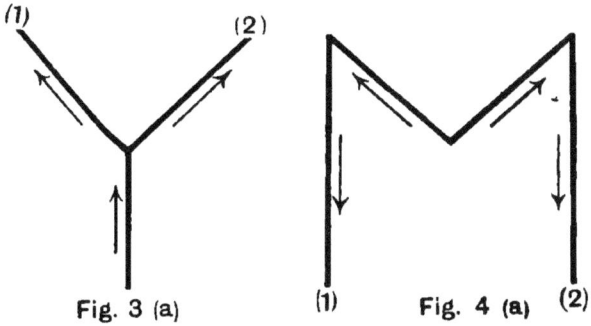

Fig. 3 (a)   Fig. 4 (a)

Following on from the points where the leaders (1) and (2) are stationed, "To rear, left and right oblique—file" (intersecting on centre) will make a letter "X" (Fig. 5 (a)).

"To rear, right and left oblique—file" to the points (1) and (2) and the outside strokes of the letter "H" are made, and by two or three pupils from the centre of No. 1 making a "Right—file," and two or three pupils in the centre of No. 2 file making a "Left—file" the "H" (Fig. 6 (a)) is completed.

Further letters can equally well be formed, but a few examples are now given of other outlines :—

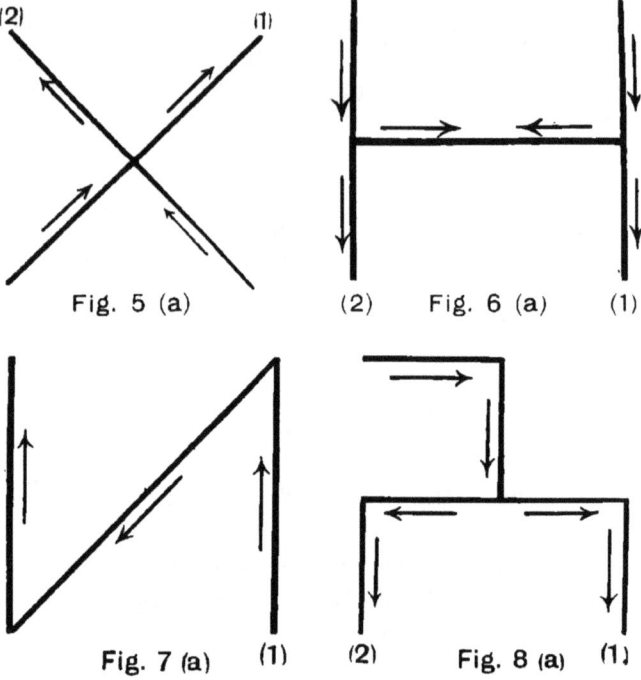

Fig. 5 (a)

(2) Fig. 6 (a) (1)

Fig. 7 (a) (1) (2) Fig. 8 (a) (1)

Starting from (1) on Fig. 7 (a) and marching in the direction of the arrow, "To rear, left oblique—file" to the corner, and then "To rear, right oblique—file" will complete the outline.

"Right—file" twice, and then "Left and right alternately—file," followed by "Right and left—file," concludes Fig. 8 (a).

Fig. 9 (a) begins with "Right and left—file," and at the point where No. 1 meets No. 2 the order is given "Forming twos, right and left—file." On reaching the centre "In twos, left and right alternately—wheel" decides Fig. 9.

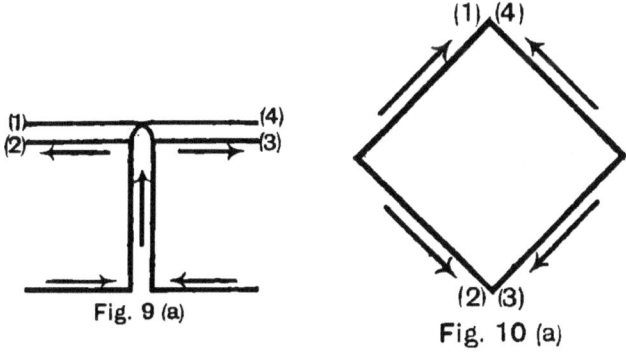

Fig. 9 (a)

Fig. 10 (a)

To form the diamond (Fig. 10 (a)) the leaders at Nos. 1 and 3 "To rear, right oblique—file," and Nos. 2 and 4 "To rear, left oblique—file."

By Nos. 1 and 3 now making a "To rear, right oblique—file," and Nos. 2 and 4 "To rear, left oblique—file," the four leaders will meet on the centre of the "cross" (Fig. 11 (a)), and by Nos. 1 and 3 making a "Right—file," and Nos. 2 and 4 a "Left—file," the "cross" will be completed.

Nos. 1 and 3 now make a "Right—file," and Nos. 2 and 4 a "Left—file," followed by "To rear, right oblique—file" and "To rear, left oblique—file" respectively in the corners, and the outline of Fig. 12 (a) is derived.

These simple figures will form a basis for endless combinations, either elementary or advanced, and whether a class consists of girls or boys, women or

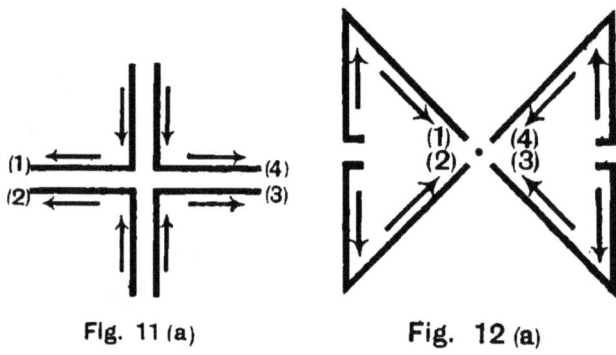

Fig. 11 (a)   Fig. 12 (a)

men, the marching can always be made suitable.

With advancement "exercises on the march" may be introduced to give further variety.

The effect may also be greatly enhanced as a display item by darkening the hall and providing each student with a lighted Chinese lantern. (In such an event "exercises on the march" would not be included.)

Where four-sided or eight-sided figures are being

formed it is advisable to work them out with a squad numbering multiples of four or eight, i.e., sixteen, twenty-four, thirty-two, etc.

Providing space permits, the larger the squad the better the effect. The following, for example, will be found very effective for a squad of sixteen or more. Beginning in single file and marching on from point (a) of Fig. 1 (b), at point (b) the order is given "Left and right alternately—file."

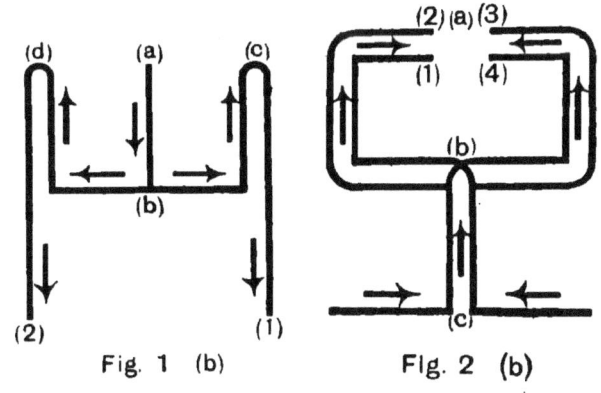

Fig. 1 (b)　　Fig. 2 (b)

The first leader always taking the first command, a further order "Left and right—file" will direct them along to (c) and (d), where "Right and left counter —file" is given, and the leaders advance to the Nos. 1 and 2, which indicate their respective order. "Right and left—file," and they will march towards (c) (Fig. 2 (b), where "Form twos, right and left—file" will take them to (b).

From here, "In twos, left and right alternately—wheel," the first pair will go left and the second pair right, with the remainder following on in similar order. "Right and left—wheel" will take them to the top corners, and "Right and left—wheel" again to the point (a).

"Form fours, right and left—wheel" and point (b) of Fig. 3 (b) is reached, while "In twos, right and left—wheel" will direct them to the sides. Nos. 1 and

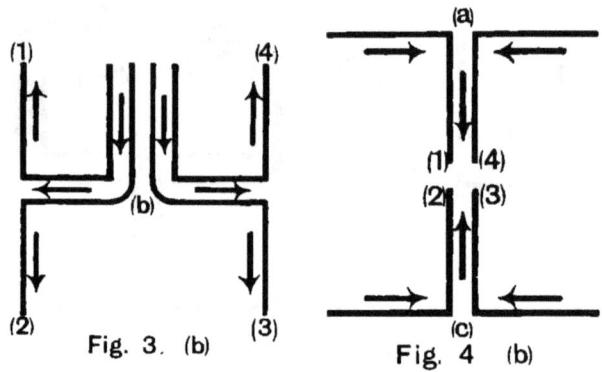

Fig. 3. (b) **Fig. 4 (b)**

3 now "Right—file" and Nos. 2 and 4 "Left—file," thus completing the figure.

A further "Right—file" by Nos. 1 and 3, and "Left—file" by Nos. 2 and 4, and (a) and (c) of Fig. 4 (b) will be reached. At this stage Nos. 1 and 4 "Form twos," likewise Nos. 2 and 3, and march on to the centre, the orders being "Form twos, Nos. 1 and 3 right—file, and Nos. 2 and 4 left—file."

Passing on to Fig. 5 (b), Nos. 1 and 3 make a "To rear, right oblique—file," and Nos. 2 and 4 "To rear, left oblique—file" to the corners, where "To rear, left oblique—file" will take them to the Nos. 1, 2, 3, and 4, which represent the numbers of the respective leaders.

"Left—file" begins (Fig. 6 (b)), and the four leaders meet on the centre, at which point "Left—file" is repeated, and they march in the direction of

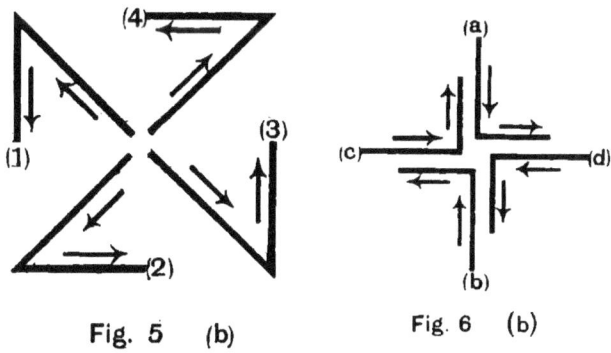

Fig. 5 (b)   **Fig. 6 (b)**

the arrows to (a), (b), (c), and (d). At these points they "Right counter—file" back to the centre. The last two orders are then repeated twice, and followed with "Left—file." This will bring the leaders at the starting points for Fig. 7 (b), and "Right—file" will direct them to the corners (1), (2), (3), and (4).

A series of right and left counter files, according to the amount of space at disposal, will complete the figure, and a "Right—file" will commence (Fig. 8 (b)). At the corners a "To rear, right oblique—file" is made, and the four leaders meet on the centre.

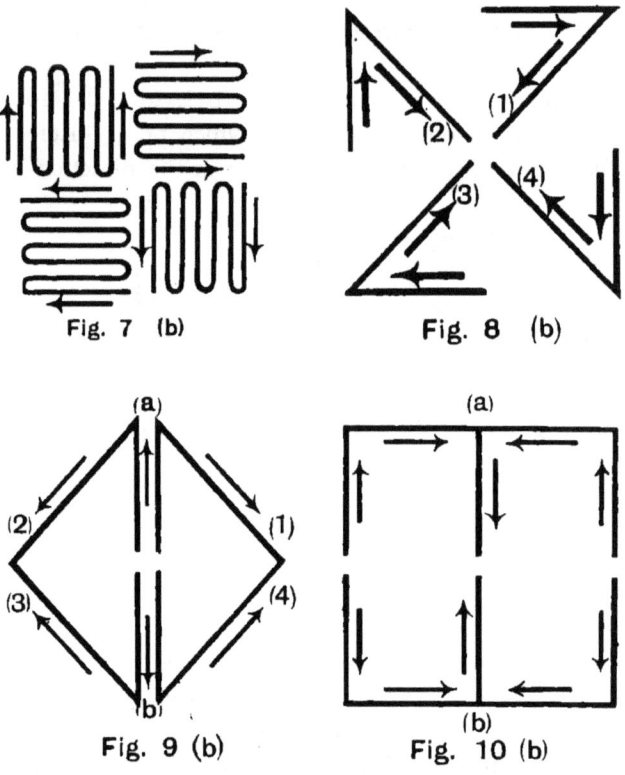

Fig. 7 (b)   Fig. 8 (b)

Fig. 9 (b)   Fig. 10 (b)

Nos. 1 and 3 now make a "To rear, right oblique—file" and form twos respectively, with Nos. 2 and 4, who make a "To rear, left oblique—file," to points (a) and (b) of Fig. 9 (b), where the odd numbers " To rear, right oblique—file," and the even numbers " To rear, left oblique—file " forming the diamond.

" To rear, left oblique—file " on the part of Nos. 1 and 3, and " To rear, right oblique—file " by Nos. 2 and 4, will take the leaders back to the corners, at which point odd numbers "Left—file" and even numbers " Right—file," meeting at (a) and (b), where

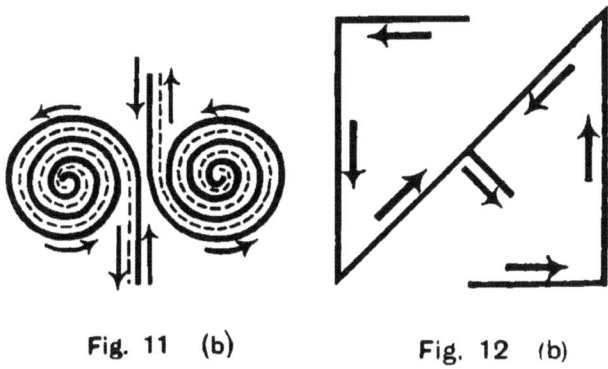

Fig. 11 (b)   **Fig. 12 (b)**

the last order being repeated single files are formed on to the centre (Fig. 10 (b)).

Branching off to the left the order is given " Form maze, left circle—file," and when in the centre of the maze " Left counter—file " will bring the leaders back to (a) and (b), the finishing points of Fig. 11 (b).

The final figure (No. 12 (b)) begins with a " Left—file," is followed by a further " Left—file " at the corners, and then " To rear, left oblique—file." The leaders now meet at the centre with No. 2, behind No. 1, and No. 4 behind No. 3, so that to return to the proper order of starting the intersecting to form single file must be done in twos. The order, therefore, is "Intersecting in twos forming single file, right and left—file." From this point the squad is marched off by the way desired.

While all the foregoing figures have been applied to ordinary marching, they can also be used for "double" marching and "exercises on the march."

TACTICAL MARCHING.

Tactical marching may be described as marching with various changes from one formation to another. It is more particularly used in military circles, where it is of inestimable value in the movement of troops.

For military purposes certain definite tactics have been laid down, together with the terms and commands for same, but the formations here set forth are for use in schools and private or public gymnasia, where the numbers are smaller and the space more confined than usually available for military work. The exercises and commands will be found to differ from those in use by the military authorities.

Consisting largely of wheeling, and changing from files to ranks, and vice versa, the more elementary movements are accomplished by turns on the march and simple wheeling in ranks. For example, "Right—turn" given to a file on the march will immediately transform it into a rank and change the direction right. In a similar manner "Left—turn" will convert a rank into a file and cause a change in direction left.

Wheeling has already been described in a previous chapter, but while the minor forms are quite easy, some of the more advanced types require a considerable amount of training to execute in good style.

For forming twos, threes, or fours on the march the file should be numbered off accordingly. If it is desired to form twos with the even numbers on the right (left), the order is given. "On the right (left) form—twos." To do this the odd numbers mark time two steps, while the even numbers step obliquely forward to the right (left) to the side of odd numbers, and both march forward together.

To form threes to the right (left) of No. 1, that number marks time the necessary steps, which in the ordinary circumstances of spacing would be three,

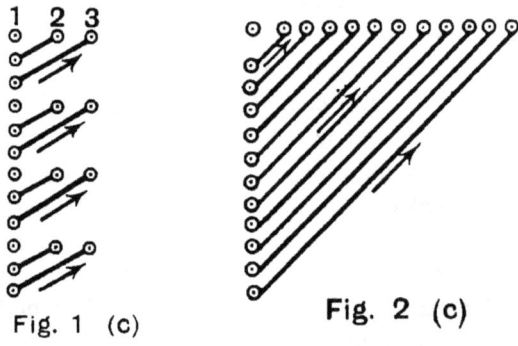

Fig. 1 (c)   Fig. 2 (c)

while No. 2 takes two steps, marking time one, and No. 3 three steps obliquely to right (left), all marching forward in line, dressing by the left (right) (see Fig. 1 (c)). The command for this would be "On the right (left) form—threes."

The whole file may form up on the right (left) in this way on the order "On the right (left) form —line" (see Fig. 2 (c)), but if the squad is a large one it is liable to become very irregular.

To achieve the same result the file may be turned to the right (left) and a "Forward (quarter) left (right)—wheel," described as in Fig. 3 (c).

A long rank may be changed into several shorter ones, and the direction altered by Nos. 2, 3, and 4 wheeling around No. 1. In Fig. 4 (c) the rank is marching forward in the direction of the arrows, and on the order "In fours forward (quarter) left—wheel" the long rank is divided up into fours, and takes a

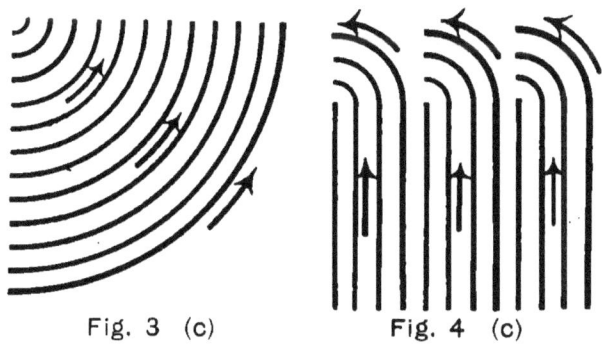

Fig. 3 (c)   Fig. 4 (c)

direction immediately to the left of the original one.

After making the "wheel" the three ranks are in what is known as "column" order.

Fig. 5 (c) shows a squad in column of fours, i.e., in ranks of fours, with a distance between each rank equal to the width of a rank.

On the command "On the right (left) form—line," one line will be formed by the leading rank marking time while the three rear ranks turn one-eighth to the right (left) and march diagonally forward at an angle of 45 degrees from the original direction. When each rank is in line with the leading rank it makes a one-eighth left (right) turn and marks time until the order is given "By the left (right)—forward," when the whole line advances dressing accordingly.

From the same starting position as in Fig. 5 (c) one line is formed facing a flank by each rank of fours

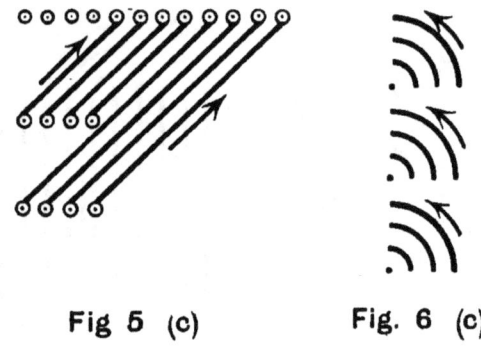

Fig 5 (c)   Fig. 6 (c)

simultaneously making a "forward (quarter) left (right)—wheel," Fig. 6 (c).

The direction of a whole rank may be changed as in Fig. 3 (c) by wheeling, or it may be changed by each student turning consecutively.

The order for this is "To right (left) change—rank," and it is carried out by the student on the extreme left (right) turning sharply to the right (left), and each successive student following consecutively with each successive step, as per Fig. 7 (c), the dotted lines representing the change.

To the order "As numbered, step forward—march," another variation may be produced from a rank, and an oblique rank formed by each student stepping forward a number of steps according to numerical order in the squad as in Fig. 8 (c), and then by turning three-eighths to the right, a single file is formed in an oblique direction.

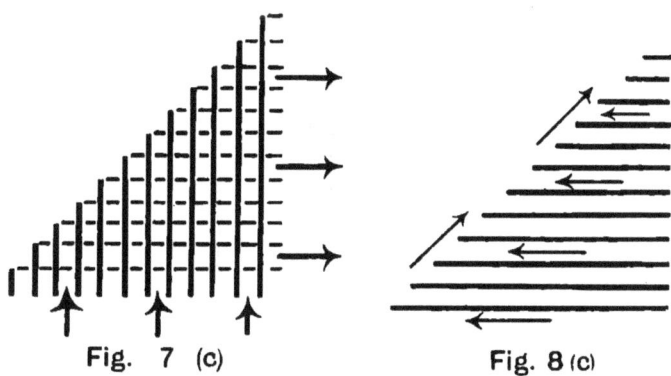

Fig. 7 (c)   Fig. 8 (c)

A further means of forming a rank from a file is as follows:—"By side and forward stepping on the left (right) form—line." With a squad of 16 (or any other number) in file with No. 1 in front, Nos. 2 to 16 inclusive take one step sideways to the left (right) and one step forward.

This will bring No. 2 at the side of No. 1. Nos. 3 to 16 then take a further step sideways to left (right) and another step forward, which places No. 3 at the side of Nos. 2 and 1.

By repeating this the whole squad will finally form up on the left (right) of No. 1 in rank order. (See Fig. 9 (c)). It is a slow process with a big squad, and will need an amount of practice to do well, but it is very effective.

Combinations of these few movements alone permit of almost endless tactics, and to give an example

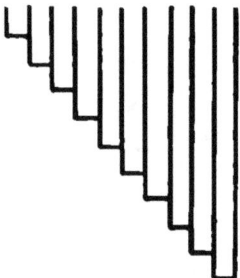

Fig. 9 (c)

of how they can be put into operation the following evolutions will serve as an illustration.

Assume a file of 16—numbered in fours—is marching in the direction of (a) Fig. 1 (d). On the command "On the right form—fours," Nos. 2, 3, and 4 will take up the positions indicated by the oblique lines and march forward in fours, taking care to keep the correct distance between the ranks. The next order is

"Backwards (quarter) left—wheel," on which No. 4 will remain on the spot making a (quarter) left turn by a series of four short steps, while Nos. 3, 2, and 1 wheel around backwards as in Fig. 2 (d).

When again in one long rank "By the left—forward" will take the rank across in the direction of the arrows in Fig. 3 (d).

At a given point "Left—turn" will change the

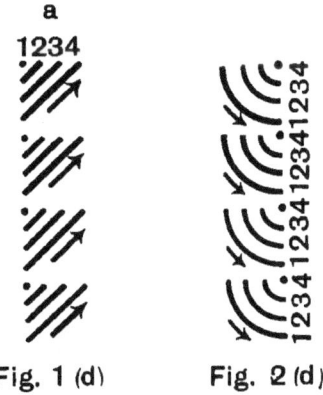

Fig. 1 (d)   Fig. 2 (d)

rank into a single file, and then "In fours, left—file" will direct the files as in Fig. 4 (d), with Nos. 1 leading. A further "Left—file" will make one single file with the order the same as at the beginning.

"Mark—time," followed by "Left—turn" and "In eights, forward, (quarter) left—wheel," will describe Fig. 5 (d).

Dividing now into fours, "In circle, complete left—

wheel" will form four circles as outlined in Fig. 6 (d). Linking up again into eights, "In circle, half left—wheel," and the squad will march as indicated

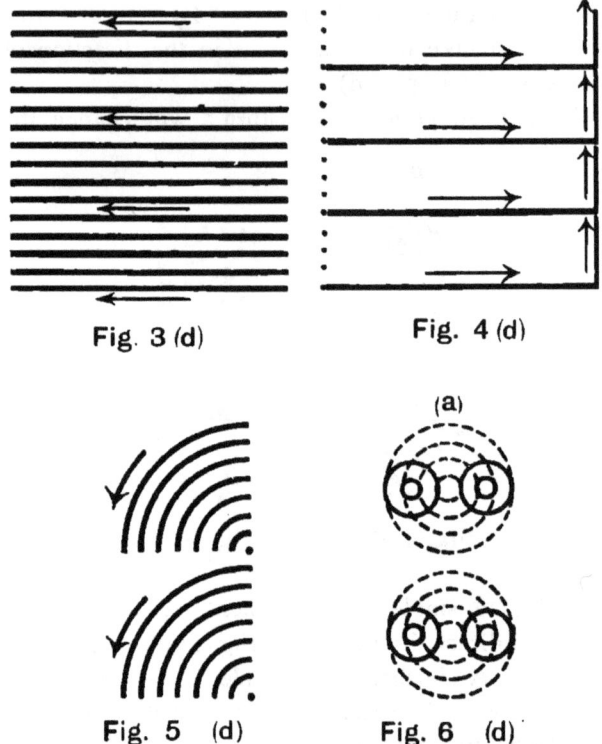

Fig. 3 (d)   Fig. 4 (d)

Fig. 5 (d)   Fig. 6 (d)

by the dotted lines and face in the direction of (a).

With two ranks of eight, numbered as in Fig. 7 (d), "Forward, quarter left—wheel" will once more make a rank of 16, and on "Right—turn" it will assume a single file.

"Right—file" now leads along the top line of Fig. 8 (d), and "By right turning, form—fours" the ranks march on to the centre, where "In twos, left and right—wheel" takes them out to the sides. Here Nos. 1 and 3 make a "Left—file," and Nos. 2 and 4 a "Right—file. (See Fig. 8 (d)).

"Odd numbers left, and even numbers right—

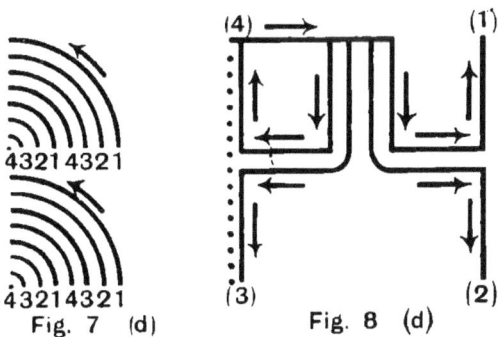

Fig. 7 (d)   Fig. 8 (d)

turn" will take the ranks in the direction of the arrows in Fig. 9 (d).

Nos. 1 and 3 now make a "Backwards, quarter right —wheel," and Nos. 2 and 4 a "Backwards, quarter left—wheel," after which they again march forward, as shown by the dotted lines in Fig. 10 (d), where "Odd numbers right and even numbers left—turn."

"To rear, odd numbers right and even numbers left oblique—file" in the corners, and the four files march on to the centre, where "Forming twos, to rear, odd numbers left, and even numbers right oblique—file," the Fig. 11 (d) is completed.

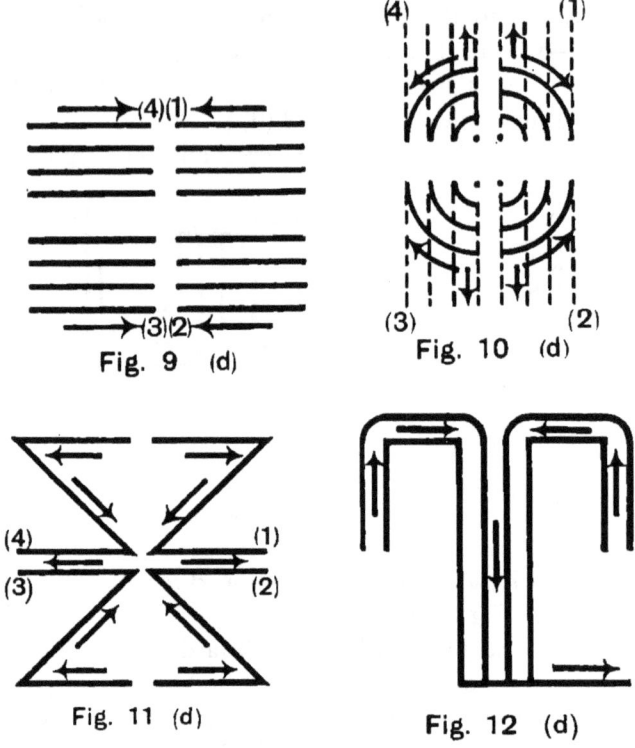

Fig. 9 (d)

Fig. 10 (d)

Fig. 11 (d)

Fig. 12 (d)

"Nos. 1 and 2 left, and Nos. 3 and 4 right—wheel" and Fig. 12 is commenced, this order being repeated at the top, and again to form fours. At the bottom, by left turning in fours, single file is formed in the original order.

Tactical marching in double rank is slightly more complicated than in single rank, and to be effective requires a fairly large squad. With 32 some good results may be obtained, and this number has been selected for the evolutions which follow:—

The squad having lined up in two ranks, (a) front and (b) rear, it is divided into two sections of 16, each numbered off from 1 to 8, the rear rank being

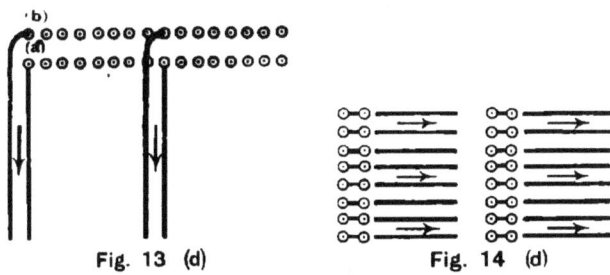

Fig. 13 (d)   Fig. 14 (d)

two paces behind and taking the same number as the front rank. The order "Right—turn," followed by "Sections, left wheel, quick—march," will take the sections in double file in the direction of the arrows on Fig. 13 (d). "Left—turn" will change them into double ranks, and alter the direction to the left as in Fig. 14 (d).

On the command "Form—fours" the odd numbers will mark time two counts while the even numbers step obliquely backward to the right of odd numbers, continuing on in fours. "Right—turn" followed by "Left—wheel," and Fig. 15 (d) is completed.

"Form twos" by odd numbers marking time two counts, and even numbers stepping obliquely back-

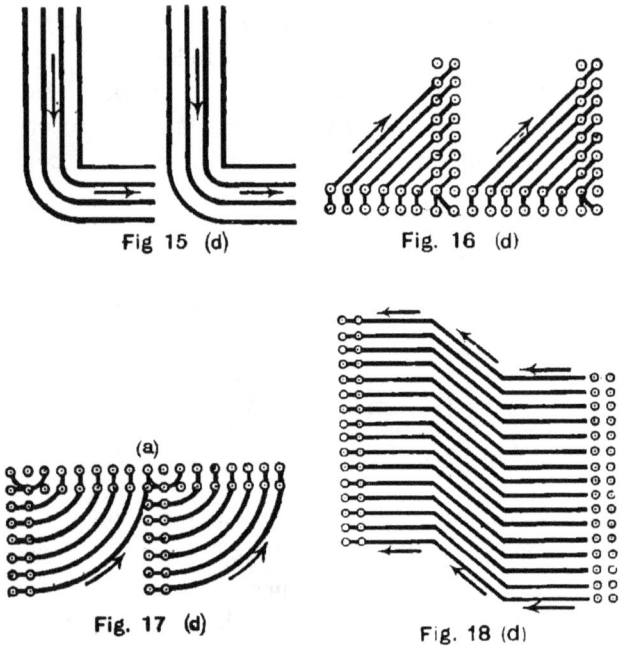

Fig 15 (d)   Fig. 16 (d)

Fig. 17 (d)   Fig. 18 (d)

ward behind odd numbers and then "Sections, on the left form—line" Fig. 16 (d) is described. "By the left —forward" and the squad will march forward in column of sections.

"Sections, left—wheel" and the squad will return

to double rank facing (a).   "Right—turn" will change the ranks into files moving to the right.

"Right—wheel" and a further "Right—turn" will begin Fig. 18 (d), the first arrow indicating the direction of the marching. "One-eighth right—turn," and the second arrow points the way, and "One-eighth left—turn" the third.

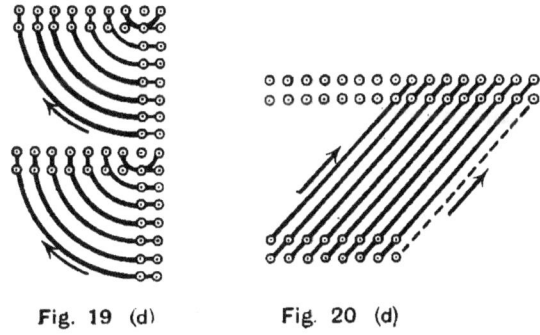

Fig. 19 (d)   Fig. 20 (d)

"Sections, right—wheel" and column of sections is formed as in Fig. 19 (d). "Squad, on the right form —line" and two ranks are again assumed with the rear rank in front, Fig. 20 (d). On "Right about— turn" the squad will be in the same order as starting.

ORNAMENTAL MARCHING.

The question is sometimes asked—What is the difference between *ornamental* and *figure* marching? A definite answer to such a query is not easy to furnish, as the line of demarcation is very indistinctly pronounced. It has been mentioned that in the category of *figure* marching the formation of stars, crosses, diamonds, letters, and in fact, any distinct outline may be included, but in so far as these also have an "ornamental" effect they may be included under this heading as well.

Ornamental marching, however, has still a wider sphere, in that it takes in any form of marching which has a spectacular effect, so that the production of various outlines may be combined with modified tactical marching, or even with exercises on the march.

It is, therefore, apparent that it is possible to bring several grades of marching under the present heading, thus presenting a very large area.

There should be no misapprehension that "ornamental" or any of the other types of spectacular marching are simply useful for their pleasing effect. This, of course, has its value, but experience proves that it is attractive to students and arouses enthusiasm and interest. These are features which must be reckoned with in physical training, for, although this training may be compulsory during school life it ends on completion of that life unless the student has found some attraction in it, and it is patent to anyone that the training of the body should not cease then any more than the training of the mind.

The psychological effect is not all, for there is a decided physical value, as explained in the early pages of this work. One may go so far as to say that a physical training lesson is incomplete without marching, and the necessity for giving this branch of exercise careful study cannot be too strongly emphasised.

Sufficient preliminaries have already been submitted of the groups comprising the sub-divisions of "ornamental" marching, and how these may be utilised and combined will be seen from the following further illustrations.

In this series it is assumed that the marching is being performed in a large room, hall, or playground, and is confined to an imaginary square.

With children it would be advisable to have the corners marked in some way, and, if practicable, the centre and diagonals also.

As to how many of the sets will be within the range of the pupils is left to the discretion of the teacher, but if two or three figures only are taken at a time and gradually connected up, there is no reason why the whole should not be mastered, and it will then supply a very effective item for a display.

As in the case of some of the other marches, the squad should be divisible by four to get the best effect, and, if possible, there should be sixteen or more pupils.

Having lined up and numbered off in fours the file advances in the direction of (a) (Fig. 1 (e)), and in the corner executes a "To rear, left oblique—file," marching diagonally across to (b), and there making a "To rear, right oblique—file" to (c).

Taking up Fig. 2 (e) at (c) a "Right—file," followed by a further "Right—file" at (a), and the point

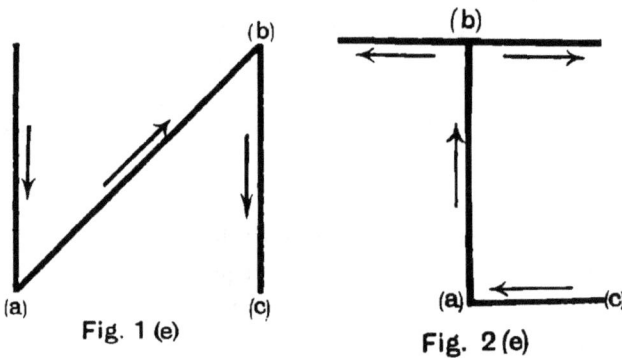

Fig. 1 (e)   Fig. 2 (e)

(b) is reached, when "Left and right alternately—file" is given. Arriving at the top corners, "Left and right—file" (Leader No. 1 taking the first command, and No. 2 the second), and the direction along the sides is traversed. "Left and right—turn" now changes the two files into ranks, and they march inwards towards each other as in Fig. 3 (e). "Right and left—turn" will make two files, or a number of ranks of twos with the leaders at (a). "Right and left—file" will direct them to the bottom corners, and "Right and left—file" again, along the sides. Half distance up the last order is repeated, and the leaders meet on the centre of Fig. 4 (e), where "Form twos, left and right—file" will take them along to (b). "In twos, left and right alternately—wheel" will complete the figure.

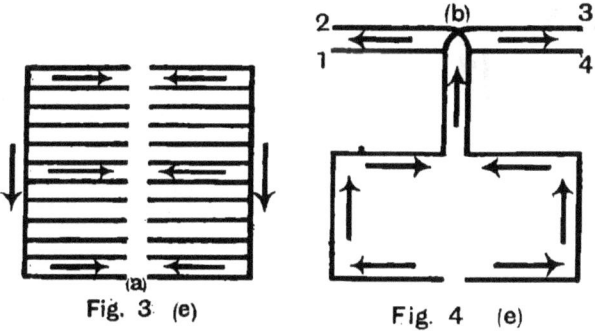

Fig. 3 (e)   Fig. 4 (e)

Fig. 5 (e) begins with "Left and right—wheel," and half way down the sides a further "Left and right—wheel" will bring the four leaders on to the centre. "Forming twos, odd numbers left, even numbers right—file," and the respective leaders will arrive at the points marked 1, 2, 3, and 4. "To rear odd numbers left, even numbers right oblique—file" will give the diamond on Fig. 6 (e), and at " To rear, odd numbers right, even numbers left oblique—file" the leaders march along the sides to the corners, where

"Odd numbers right, even numbers left—turn." The four ranks then march forward as in Fig. 7 (e), when "Backward, odd numbers quarter right, even numbers quarter left—wheel," as in Fig. 8 (e)

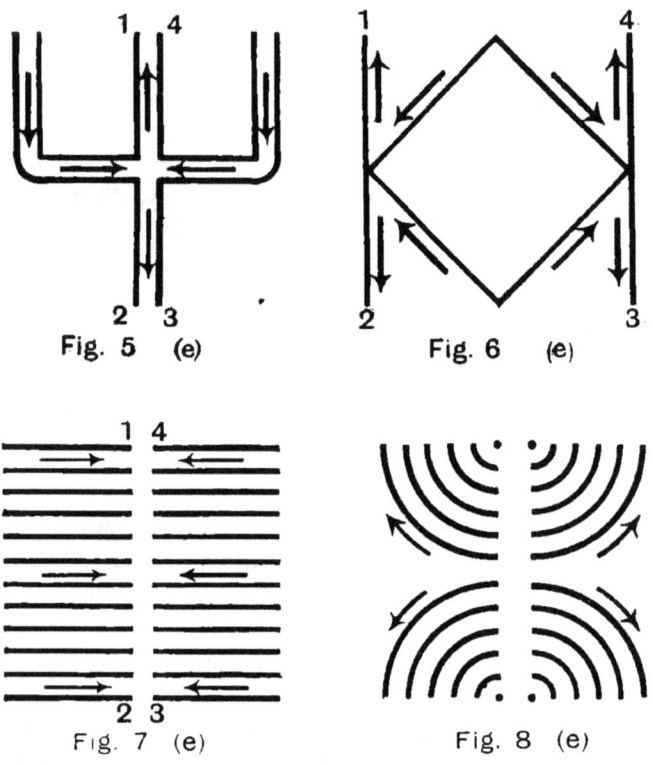

Fig. 5 (e)   Fig. 6 (e)

Fig. 7 (e)   Fig. 8 (e)

At the completion of the quarter wheel, "Odd numbers left, and even numbers right—turn," and "Form twos, odd numbers right, and even numbers left—file," making the first part of Fig. 9 (e). On reaching the centre " To rear, odd numbers right, even numbers left oblique—file " takes the leaders obliquely back to the corners, where each of the four files " To rear, left oblique—file." When four or more steps have been taken in this direction, according to the number of students in each file, " Left—turn " is

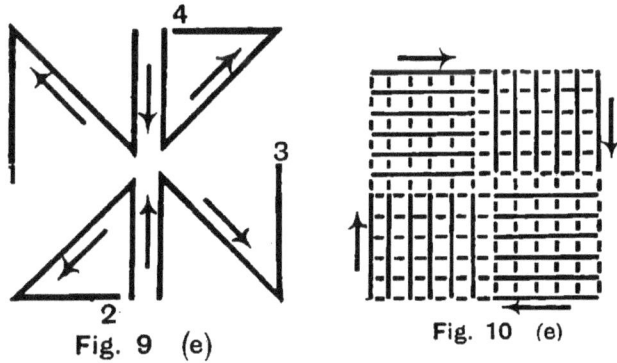

Fig. 9 (e)   Fig. 10 (e)

given, and an effective quadrangular march is performed by each rank marching across to the opposite corner. (See Fig. 10 (e)). At the corner the order " Backward, quarter right—wheel " will take the leaders backward through a quarter circle, and the rank will be ready to march forward again to the next corner. The command " Backwards, quarter right—wheel" may be repeated three times, so that the whole four corners are covered (Fig. 11 (e)). At the end of the last quarter wheel "Right—turn" will furnish four files with the leaders in front. "**Left—file**" will then bring them along the dotted lines of Fig. 12 (e) with the respective leaders on the places numbered 1, 2, 3, and 4. "Left—turn" and "In circle (complete) left—wheel" and the four circles are described, and the leaders are back again on the numbers shown in that figure. Each rank now makes a "Forward

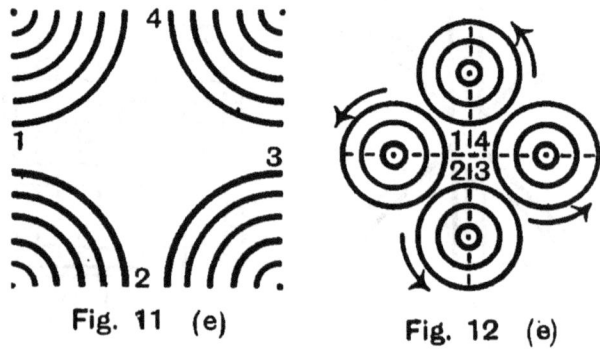

Fig. 11 (e) Fig. 12 (e)

(complete) right—wheel," which disposes of Fig. 13 (e), and the leaders will still be as in Fig. 12 (e). "Right—turn" and then "Intersect, forming two files, to rear, odd numbers right, even numbers left oblique—file" and Fig. 14 (e) makes its entry with the two files marching from the centre to the corners, at which "To rear, right oblique—file" is given for the march along the sides.

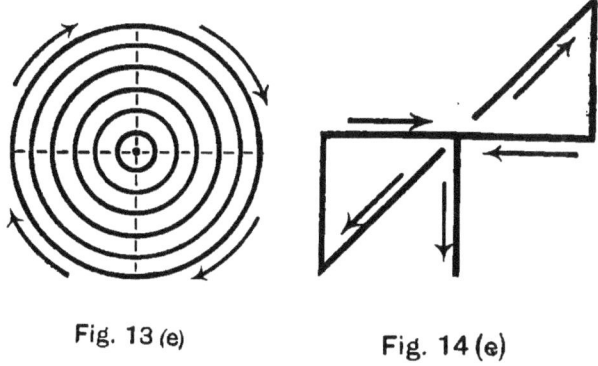

Fig. 13 (e)   Fig. 14 (e)

At half distance " Right—file " will cause the two leaders to meet on the centre, where " Intersect in twos, forming single file, right and left—file " the final stage is reached.

www.ingramcontent.com/pod-product-compliance
Lightning Source LLC
Chambersburg PA
CBHW060213050426
42446CB00013B/3067